YOUR KNOWLEDGE HAS VALUE

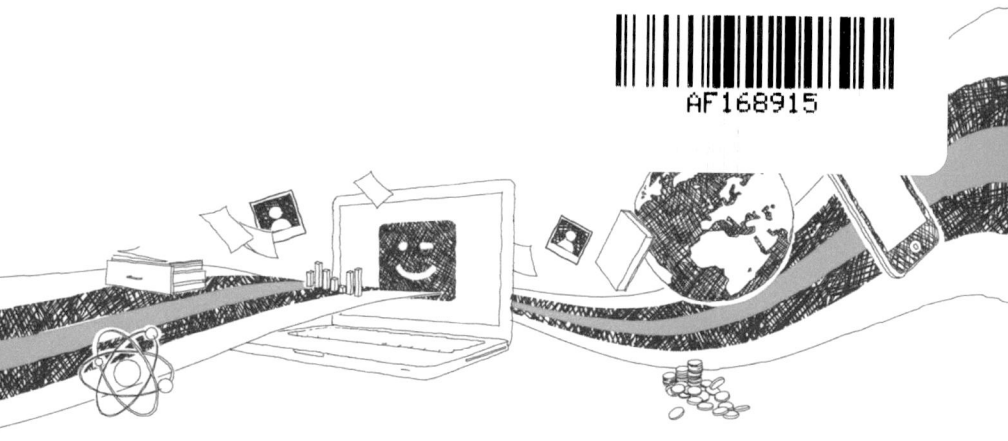

- We will publish your bachelor's and master's thesis, essays and papers

- Your own eBook and book - sold worldwide in all relevant shops

- Earn money with each sale

Upload your text at www.GRIN.com and publish for free

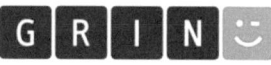

Bibliographic information published by the German National Library:

The German National Library lists this publication in the National Bibliography; detailed bibliographic data are available on the Internet at http://dnb.dnb.de .

This book is copyright material and must not be copied, reproduced, transferred, distributed, leased, licensed or publicly performed or used in any way except as specifically permitted in writing by the publishers, as allowed under the terms and conditions under which it was purchased or as strictly permitted by applicable copyright law. Any unauthorized distribution or use of this text may be a direct infringement of the author s and publisher s rights and those responsible may be liable in law accordingly.

Imprint:

Copyright © 2016 GRIN Verlag, Open Publishing GmbH
Print and binding: Books on Demand GmbH, Norderstedt Germany
ISBN: 9783668575653

This book at GRIN:

https://www.grin.com/document/380826

Patrick Kimuyu

Diet and Disease in America

GRIN Publishing

GRIN - Your knowledge has value

Since its foundation in 1998, GRIN has specialized in publishing academic texts by students, college teachers and other academics as e-book and printed book. The website www.grin.com is an ideal platform for presenting term papers, final papers, scientific essays, dissertations and specialist books.

Visit us on the internet:

http://www.grin.com/

http://www.facebook.com/grincom

http://www.twitter.com/grin_com

DIET AND DISEASE IN AMERICA

Name: Patrick K. Kimuyu

Diet has become one of the principal causes of the emerging diseases, especially the so-called Non-communicable Diseases (NCD's) among the global population. Currently, most countries have experienced transient nutrition transition, owing to changes in lifestyle and the availability of dietary products. Globally, it seems most people have abandoned their traditional diet and adopted modern eating habits, which tend to favor the consumption of dietary fats, especially from animal products (Boushey, Coulston & Ferruzzi, 2012). In contrast, the highest percentage of the global population has reduced the consumption of a vegetarian diet such as vegetables and fruits; instead, most people have increased high-fat diet intake (WHO, 2003).

Surprisingly, the ultimate result for the transient nutrition transition among the global population is the unprecedented increase of mortality rates related to Non-communicable diseases such as cancer, cardiovascular diseases and diabetes.

In America, diet related diseases have become an immense public healthcare problem to the healthcare system because; diet related diseases have assumed upward trends. Currently, Non-communicable diseases have become the leading cause of deaths, in the United States of America (Hospedales, 2011). These trends can be attributed to the excessive consumption of animal dietary products because; biomedical research has identified the harmful effects of animal dietary products on human health. Animal dietary products have been found to cause numerous health problems to humans, although they provide essential nutritional requirements to the human body but, excessive consumption increases the risk of suffering from diet related diseases. On the other hand, vegetables and fruits have been found to be reliable remedies to Non-communicable diseases. Therefore, this essay will give an overview of the diet and disease correlation.

Currently, it has emerged that an individual's health status is determined by the type of diet an individual consumes. The current trends of excessive consumption of animal dietary products explain the reason as to why Non-communicable diseases, commonly referred to as 'lifestyle diseases' have become the most prevalent among the American population. Nutritional research indicates that animal dietary products contain high amounts of unsaturated fats, which is believed to be the principal cause of health problems to most people (Boyle & Long, 2008). These fats are believed to lead to incidences of obesity, cardiovascular diseases, cancer and diabetes.

Trends in Dietary Supply of Fat (g per capita per day)

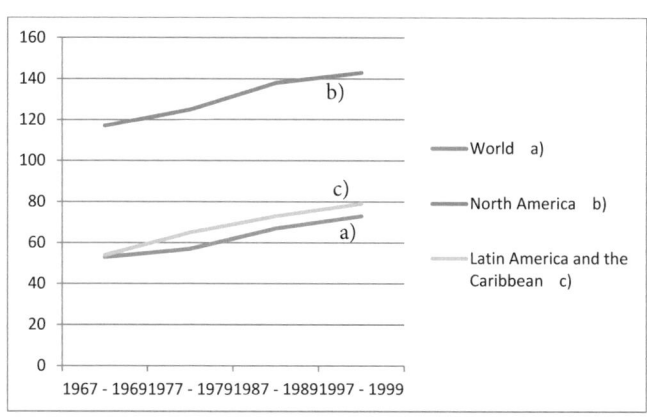

Source: WHO, 2003

In America, obesity has become the most prevalent Non-communicable disease with more than half of the US population being obese. Recent epidemiological reports show that 35.9% of adults are obese, whereas, children aged 6-11 years and adolescents account for 18.0% and 18.4%, respectively. Further reports reveal that, in 2010, 12.1% of children aged between 2 to 5 years, in the US are obese (CDC, 2012). As a result, the US Healthcare system experiences an enormous burden from obesity.

Obesity refers to a health condition in which an individuals' body weight exceeds the required healthy limits. In other words, individuals whose Body Mass Index exceeds 29.5 in value are considered to be obese. In general, obesity is believed to be caused by a transient change of lifestyle from physical activity to a sedentary lifestyle accompanied with excessive intake of carbohydrates and animal fats. It has been found that excessive intake of animal fats leads to the accumulation of fat in the body of an individual, which are stored in fat deposits, usually around the waist (Boushey, Coulston & Ferruzzi, 2012). These fats are hardly consumed for oxidative respiration to generate energy for physical activity and other biological functions in the body. As a result, fat tissues are stacked with fat layers, leading to a rapid weight increase of an individual. Continued intake of animal products, which are rich in fats, leads to excessive accumulation of fat deposits, hence an increase in one's Body Mass Index value. Ordinarily, excessive accumulation of fats in the body is manifested by the rapid enlargement of the waistline.

In most cases, obese individuals experience difficulties in locomotion due to the excessive weight gain, leading to the malfunctioning of the leg joints and muscles. However, it is worth noting that, excessive weight gain among the obese people has been found to cause other health conditions. Some of the health conditions related to obesity diabetes and arthritis. Arthritis occurs due to the excessive accumulation of body weight, which burdens the leg joints during movement. In most case, bone cartilage lining the joints wear out, leading to increased friction between the bones and, this is manifested by pain within the knee joints during movement. Therefore, obesity causes the highest percentage of immobility among obese people.

On the other hand, animal fats increase the risk of diabetes among the obese people. Biomedical research reveals that, most animal dietary products contain high levels of unsaturated fats, which are not utilized in the body for respiratory activities; instead, they are deposited in the lipid bi-layer, which forms the cell membrane; thus, interfering with the functioning of the body cells. As a result, permeability of nutritional macromolecules such as glucose and proteins is adversely impaired, leading to the so-called glucose resistance by the body cells. As a result, glucose and other simple sugars accumulate in the blood stream leading to a condition referred to as hyperglycemia (high blood sugar), which in turn, leads to the onset of diabetes.

Currently, diabetes, in the U.S is assuming upward trends with 25.8 million people among the US population being diabetic. Recent epidemiological results indicate that, in 2010, 18.8 million people were diagnosed with diabetes, whereas 7.0 million remain undiagnosed. In general, more than 8.3% of the U.S population is suffering from diabetes (CDC, 2011). Further epidemiological reports indicate that, an estimation of 79 million people, in the US are pre-diabetes, whereas the number of new cases among the population aged 20 years and above, in 2010, was 1.9 million (American Diabetes Association, 2011).

On the other hand, the consumption of animal dietary products has been found to increase the risk of cardiovascular diseases because; unsaturated dietary fats are believed to contribute significantly to the onset of the diseases. Some of the cardiovascular diseases related to the excessive intake of dietary fats include the heart disease, hypertension and stroke.

In general, animal dietary products contain high levels of unsaturated fatty acids, cholesterol and Low Density Lipoprotein (LDL), which are believed to cause the harmful health effects in the human body (Boyle & Long, 2008).

For instance, hypertension is caused by excessive accumulation of animal-derived fats in the blood circulatory system, leading to the deposition of fats on the walls of the blood arteries. As a result, the lumen of blood vessels narrows, causing resistance in blood flow. The systolic pressure of blood forces blood through the narrow lumen leading to an unprecedented increase of blood pressure within the blood vessels. This condition is manifested by the rise of an individual's blood pressure (BP), beyond the expected normal limits. Ordinarily, blood pressure of a normal individual ranges between 120 mmHg and 130mmHg with regard to the systolic pressure. Therefore, blood pressure rates above 130mmHg are usually harmful and, individuals whose systolic blood pressure exceeds 130mmHg are referred to as hypertensive. Currently, about 50% of the American population is at a risk of suffering from hypertension (Boushey, Coulston & Ferruzzi, 2012). Therefore, it is predicted that incidence rates for stroke, heart attack and kidney failure among the U.S population will increase by two-folds in the next two decades. Surprisingly, heart disease and stroke are related to hypertension and their causes are relatively the same. In regard to heart disease and stroke, excessive fat deposition on the arterial walls leads to eventual blockage or rapture of the blood vessels. Heart disease is caused by the accumulation of cholesterol and other fats on the coronary arteries, which innervate the heart muscles, forming 'plaques' (Boyle & Long, 2008). Formation of plaques leads to the clogging of the arteries; thus, supply of nutrients to the heart muscles becomes interrupted. Blockage of the coronary arteries causes cessation of the heart muscle functioning, which in turn, results into a heart attack or failure, hence death.

On the other hand, stroke is caused by the formation of plaques in the brain vessels; thus, interfering with the function of the brain. In most cases, blood capillaries in the brain are clogged by the fat deposits, leading to the death of the concerned brain region. Blood capillaries are also believed to rupture due to the excessive pressure from the arteries, owing to the narrowing of the capillary lumen. The ultimate result of the brain's capillary blockage and rupture is the death of some brain cells, leading to the unprecedented impairment of the brain function (Boyle & Long, 2008). Therefore, body organs, which are controlled by the damaged region of the brain, are paralyzed and, this is the onset of a health condition known as stroke.

Moreover, diet has been found to increase the risk of certain cancers. Biomedical research reveals that, high-fat diet, especially from animal sources increases the risk of cancer. For instance, the causes colon cancer and breast cancer are believed to be diet related. Currently, colon cancer is the leading cause of mortality among cancer patients, in the US and, breast cancer has emerged the leading cancer killer among the American women (Sharlin, 2010).

The pathophysiology of breast cancer has not been studies extensively but, clinical trials reveal that, the intake of high-fat diet plays significant roles in causing breast cancer among women. Animal dietary products contain high levels of Low Density Lipoprotein (LDL), which reacts with Reactive Oxygen Species (ROS); thus, interfering with the cellular activities in the cell nucleus (Sharlin, 2010). This results into irregular cell division in various parts of the body forming cancerous growths or tumor cells.

In regard to colon cancer, the high levels of fat in animal dietary products cause unprecedented retention of food within the digestive tract. As a result, microbial flora in the colon releases carcinogenic toxins, which in turn, causes tumors of the colon walls (Bendich & Deckelbaum, 2010). One of the most harmful pathogenic bacteria is called Helicobacter pylori and, it inhabits the gastro-intestinal tract of humans.

However, nutritional approaches have emerged to be the most appropriate remedy for most lifestyle diseases. It has been found that, change of unhealthy eating habits plays a significant role in preventing diet related diseases such as obesity, diabetes, cancer and heart diseases. For instance, a dietary regime rich in vegetables and fruits has proven to safeguard people from Non-communicable diseases. Vegetables and fruits do not contain cholesterol and unsaturated fatty acids; thus, they do not cause health risks to people; instead, they contain protective nutritional components, which enhance the body's immune response towards diseases. For instance, vegetables and fruits are known to contain phyto-chemicals, which act as anti-oxidants. Therefore, anti-oxidants such as vitamin E and Lycopene aid in removing Reactive Oxygen Species (ROS), which are responsible for causing cancer from the body (Bendich & Deckelbaum, 2010).

Conclusively, it is blatantly true that, a vegetarian diet holds promise in prevention of Non-communicable diseases such as cancer, diabetes and heart diseases. Vegetarian diet contains all the essential nutrients required by the body for normal functioning. It is true to assert that, in the 21st Century, an individuals' healthy status is depended on the dietary portions in the plate, especially with regard to lifestyle related diseases. Therefore, the ever rising prevalence trends of chronic diseases such as cancer, heart disease, obesity and its related health conditions can be reversed by the adoption of a vegetarian diet (Boushey, Coulston & Ferruzzi, 2012). However, animal dietary servings are required for the supply of some of the most essential nutritional requirements; nevertheless, high-fat diets should be avoided. A vegetarian diet is the most appropriate alternative for preventing the prevalence of most diseases among the American population and the world at large.

References

American Diabetes Association (2011). *Diabetes Statistics.* Retrieved from http://www.diabetes.org/diabetes-basics/diabetes-statistics/

Bendich, A. & Deckelbaum, R. (2010). *Preventive Nutrition: The Comprehensive Guide for Health Professionals.* New York, NY: Springer.

Boushey, C., Coulston, A. & Ferruzzi, M. (2012). *Nutrition in the Prevention and Treatment of Disease.* Waltham, MA: Academic Press.

Boyle, M. & Long, S. (2008). *Personal Nutrition.* Stamford, CT: Cengage Learning.

CDC (2011). *2011 National Diabetes Fact Sheet.* Retrieved from http://www.cdc.gov/diabetes/pubs/estimates11.htm

CDC (2012). *Obesity and Overweight.* Retrieved from http://www.cdc.gov/nchs/fastats/overwt.htm

Hospedales, C. (2011). *Global to Country Level: Perceptions and Trends in NCDs in the Americas.* Retrieved from http://www.gbchealth.org/system/documents/category_53/314/Global%20to%20Country%20Level_Perceptions%20&%20Trends%20in%20NCDs%20in%20the%20Americas_J.Hospedales.pdf?1344534649

Sharlin, S. (2010). *Life Cycle Nutrition: Evidence Based Approach.* Burlington, MA: Jones & Bartlett Publishers.

WHO (2003). *Diet, Nutrition and the Prevention of Chronic Diseases.* Retrieved from http://www.fao.org/docrep/005/AC911E/AC911E00.HTM

YOUR KNOWLEDGE HAS VALUE

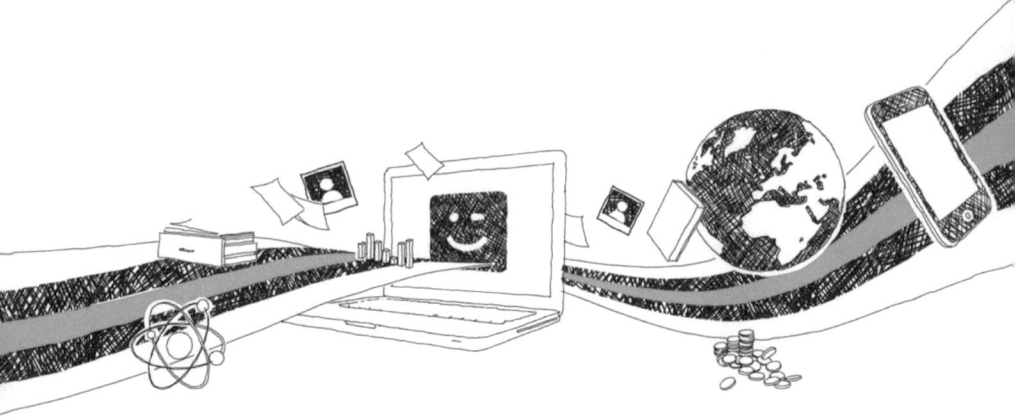

- We will publish your bachelor's and master's thesis, essays and papers

- Your own eBook and book - sold worldwide in all relevant shops

- Earn money with each sale

Upload your text at www.GRIN.com
and publish for free

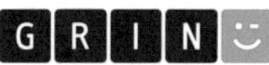